The 14 Day Carnivore Challenge

Jason Atkinson

INTRODUCTION

For years I had this dream of becoming a published author. I imagined that one day I would meet someone in passing who would casually ask what I did for a living to which I would reply "I'm a health coach" and then I would hand this person a card or give them a link directing him or her to a website where they would be able to purchase my books, audio programs and other coaching materials along with all the free content like videos, articles and podcasts I have created over the years. Today that dream is a reality!

In 2018 I published my first book **Live Like an Athlete** and made it available on Amazon. When I received the first print edition in the mail, I was as excited as a father seeing his newborn child for the first time. As I held this tangible "proof" in my hands, the years of struggle and sacrifice that led to permanently losing 75 pounds of unhealthy bodyfat suddenly all seemed worthwhile because now I had created something that would help others to experience similar results faster and with much less time, effort and sacrifice than I endured through trial and error.

In the years since then, I've learned so much more about nutrition and discovered a vast array of new exercise techniques and key supplementation strategies that contribute to a lifestyle of fitness and overall vitality that I've decided to compile an entire series of Audiobooks, E books and print versions of my "Apex Human" series. This is the first book in the series.

The takeaway is this: Never give up, no matter how hard it gets. The idea of helping others was a huge motivator for me to achieve my own weight loss goals in the first place. If you're struggling to stay on track, keep looking ahead to a time when others will benefit from what you have learned. This just may be the extra edge you need to stay consistent. With that, I present: The 14 Day Carnivore Challenge!

CONTENTS

Acknowledgments   i

Day 1   The Pyramid Scheme   Pg 1

Day 2   The Great Reset   Pg 3

Day 3   The Protein Prescription   Pg 7

Day 4   Calorie Confusion   Pg 11

Day 5   Build and Burn   Pg 15

Day 6   The Plant Paradox   Pg 19

Day 7   You Are What You Eat   Pg 23

Day 8   Cheat Meals vs Refeeds   Pg 27

Day 9   Get In The Zone   Pg 31

Day 10   The Science of Ancestral Diets   Pg 35

Day 11   Fat For Fuel   Pg 39

Day 12   How Does a Carnivore Diet Work?   Pg 43

Day 13   Slow Poison   Pg 47

Day 14   The Real Human Diet   Pg 51

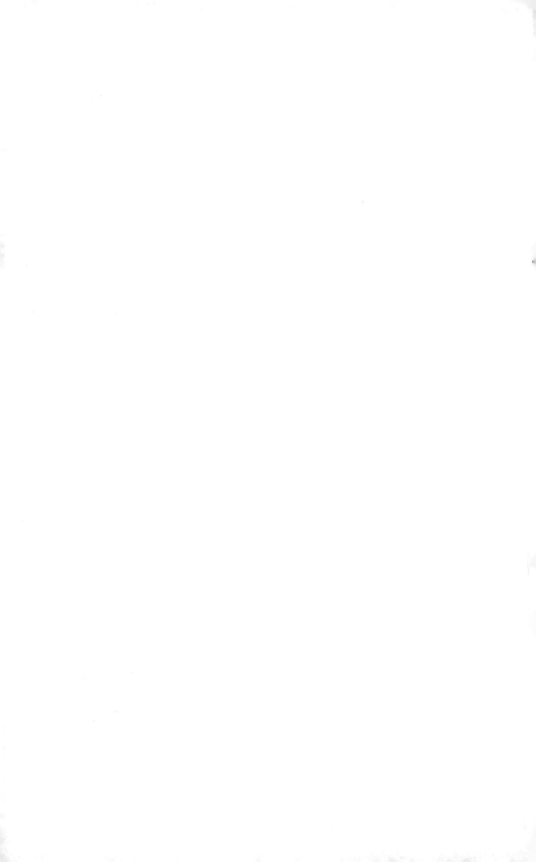

ACKNOWLEDGMENTS

I would like to acknowledge that writing a book is never a solo project. Aside from the many influencers in the health and wellness space who have helped me through an array of audiovisual and print media, I would like to acknowledge the love and support of my friends and family.

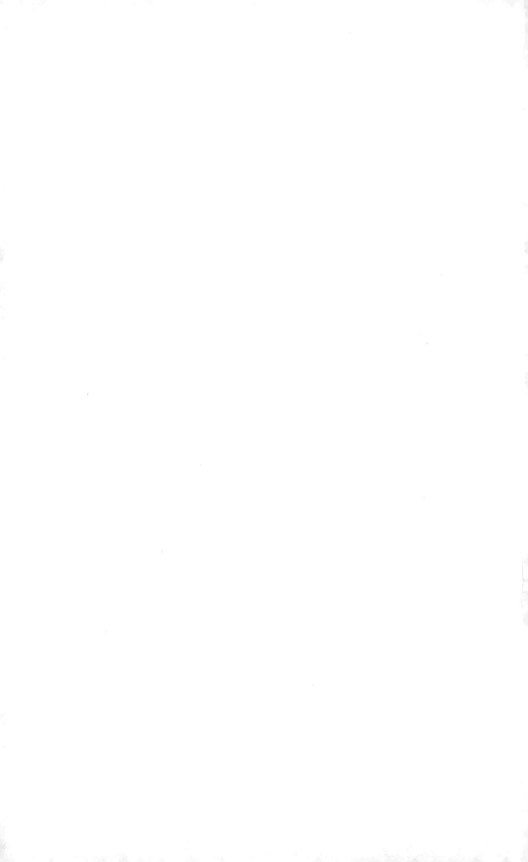

DAY 1 THE PYRAMID SCHEME

If there is a ground zero for obesity in America, it would be the original Dietary Guidelines for Americans, represented by a food pyramid. The recommendations were made under the guise of being motivated by health. However, in truth they were issued primarily with financial profit in mind. A "Food Pyramid" depicting a proper human diet should have been the exact opposite all along! Instead, low-fat fears (thanks mainly to the flimsy "research" of Dr Ancel Keys) were used to promote a grain-based diet.

You see, grains are very cheap to produce and have a long shelf life. Plus, they can be transformed into all kinds of addictive food like products by adding other cheap ingredients such as sugar, salt, high fructose corn syrup along with industrial seed oils such as soy, canola and corn.

These ingredients are highly inflammatory in the human body and wreak havoc on blood sugar and insulin. The solution to the chronic health problems our society faces is to return to a natural diet based on animal protein and avoid excess carbohydrates and refined fats especially man-made or processed ones. Fears surrounding foods like red meat and eggs based on saturated fat or dietary cholesterol content are completely unfounded. To the contrary, these are some of the most nutrient-dense foods that exist.

To this day, there is no proven link between dietary fat intake and heart disease. There is no link between dietary cholesterol intake and elevated serum-cholesterol. There is also no proof that elevated total serum cholesterol is a risk factor for heart disease or any other disease.

If you simply imagine "cutting the base off the pyramid" remember, it will still stand without the recommendations to eat a grain-based diet. These recommendations were motivated primarily by corporate greed and not human health. Food companies and other special interests put profits before people and our entire population has been paying the price ever since.

You can begin your journey towards an animal-based/ low-carb (or "carnivore") lifestyle today by reducing or eliminating grains like wheat, corn, oats and rice, and instead focusing on high-quality food like beef, eggs and salmon (to name a few)! Don't worry if it's not "perfect". Just start heading in that direction and you'll be amazed at the positive results on your health, energy as well as mental and physical well-being.

DAY 2 THE GREAT RESET

Today is the first day of a new week and it's when I usually "reset" my metabolism back to fat-burning and muscle-building/preservation mode after the weekend. Yes, this challenge is about adopting an animal-based, low-carb (a.k.a. "Carnivore") lifestyle, but today I want to discuss another Ancestral Health Principle I use, known as Intermittent Fasting.

If you're not familiar with the concept, it simply means not eating for part of the day, effectively extending your overnight "fast". Fasting is one of the oldest and most popular health practices. Every culture and religion has practiced times of restrictive food intake throughout history.

For most of our time as a species on this planet, food was not always as abundant as it is now. Therefore, we developed the ability to store excess food, primarily in the form of adipose tissue (or bodyfat), to have an energy source available when food is not around.

Our hunter-gatherer ancestors may have sometimes gone without food for several days while attempting to hunt or gather something edible.

In the modern world we've been conditioned (mostly through commercial advertising and cultural traditions) to eat frequently, usually as a response to the sensation of hunger which is actually a combination of low blood sugar and a spike in the hormone ghrelin that subsides quickly if we don't respond.

Ghrelin's job is to "remind" us to eat to protect those precious fat stores and prevent starvation. Most of us are carrying around enough stored energy in the form of fat to walk hundreds of miles or go several days without eating specifically for energy.

I'm not a fan of extended fasting but Intermittent fasting is a little different. We're already fasting 8-12 hours straight most days anyway which is why we don't starve to death in our sleep. If we don't interrupt the overnight fast with a significant intake of dietary energy (calories) especially from carbohydrate, we will continue to burn fat throughout the day.

The key with Intermittent Fasting is to do it but don't overdo it. It works best when it's the exception not the rule. It works so well; it's tempting to do it practically every day and therein lies the danger. When I first began employing this strategy, I went straight to a 20 hour fast which left me with only 1-2 meals at the end of the day to try and meet my nutrient goals.

Even though it's relatively painless, and you will be "bouncing off the walls" with energy especially if you're also restricting carbohydrates) don't fall into the trap of doing it every day. In the short term you will simply produce ketones and experience no drop in energy. However, when a food shortage becomes severe and prolonged your body enacts measures designed to keep you alive including catabolizing muscle tissue and making you feel sluggish to "slow you down" and prevent the drain on internal energy stores.

To institute an intermittent fast, just extend your regular 8-12 hour overnight fast by an additional 8-12 waking hours and be sure to follow it up with a good amount of protein and other vital nutrients. This is another case where prioritizing animal-based foods can help.

Also, you can modify your intermittent fast to incorporate a small caloric value from either protein and/or fat without interrupting the fasted state. I wouldn't consume any amount of sugar or carbohydrates since this will interrupt the fast. Unless you're trying to maximize autophagy (cellular cleanup) you could consume a very small amount of protein or fat, perhaps added to coffee or tea or maybe even a little broth.

I'm sure you have questions about this and I'm all ears. You can contact me during this challenge or anytime by visiting linktr.ee/truetransformation.coach .

Remember, this is not medical advice and I'm not a medical professional, just a guy who lost a bunch of weight who can help you do the same thing is that's what you want. While you're checking out my podcasts, videos, articles and social media posts, schedule a free consultation by phone or video chat and I'll help you get to the bottom of your health and fitness struggles once and for all.

DAY 3 THE PROTEIN PRESCRIPTION

In my line of work as a certified Health Coach, Nutritionist and Personal Trainer, I'm often asked by clients, "How much protein should I eat each day?" The answer depends on your goals. The "official" Daily Reference Intake for protein (as established by the Institute of Medicine) is only 0.8 grams of protein for every kilogram of body weight per day. (I did the math, that's .36g per pound of body weight). Using that guideline, a 200 lb individual would only "need" 75 grams of protein per day (the amount found in 3/4 lb of lean meat). For a 150 lb female that's only about 50g per day (the equivalent of one grilled chicken breast and a cup of yogurt).

While this may be adequate to prevent muscle wasting in an inactive person, it's not ideal for someone who regularly engages in heavy resistance training or other activity. As with all nutritional RDAs (Recommended Daily Allowances) this amount represents the bare minimum to sustain life and not the optimal amount needed to thrive.

The famous "one gram of protein per pound of body weight per day" formula became popular among bodybuilders and other strength athletes in the "Golden Era of Bodybuilding" during the 1960s and 1970s, as a handy way to estimate protein needs. Modern science now verifies they were onto something!

The classic bodybuilding diet was both animal-based and low-carb. Bodybuilders were the original biohackers who focused on the true "superfoods" of human nutrition like beef, eggs and cottage cheese to support their efforts in the gym.

Along with an overall lifestyle built around strength and health that included heavy resistance training and cardiovascular conditioning, the bodybuilders of the Golden Era also spent time outdoors basking in the golden sun of Venice, California near the "Mecca of Bodybuilding" the original Gold's Gym.

Of course, they occasionally ate vegetables and sometimes fruit, but starchy carbs such as rice and potatoes were not staples of the diet. They limited their carbohydrate intake to just trace amounts and kept dietary protein high most of the time. One day a week they had a "junk day" where anything was fair game including pies, ice cream, pizza, tacos and whatever else they wanted, but aside from that, it was strictly high-protein, low-carb.

A modern meta-analysis of the research concerning protein intake suggests 30-40g approximately 3-5 times per day as a good estimate for the general public engaging in moderate amounts of exercise. That's more like a total of 90-150g on the low end and 120-200g per day on the high end which correlates closely to the "one gram per pound" rule. Factors like body size, lean body mass and activity level influence the need for protein but 30-40g per meal is a reasonable starting point.

People often wonder if "too much protein" will interrupt ketosis or prevent them from entering a fat burning state. The answer is "not likely". You don't need to be in ketosis to lose weight but if you reduce carbs low enough you might actually feel better if you remove them almost completely, at least for the majority of the time. This will cause your body to produce ketones to support brain function and spare glucose stored as glycogen in the muscle to fuel your activity.

Your body can also convert protein into glucose as needed through a process known as gluconeogenesis. This comes in pretty handy when your carb intake is low, but you still engage in glycolytic (high energy demand) activity. There is no requirement for carbohydrates in human metabolism and if you eat enough protein, you don't need carbs for energy either.

The bottom line is that protein is a great regulator of appetite and is necessary for cell turnover and enzyme formation in addition to providing the raw material to recover and rebuild from intensive training. People who are interested in improving body composition should worry about not getting enough protein rather than too much.

If you want to get technical, track your intake and see what amount gives you the best appetite control and produces benefits in the gym, but an intuitive approach also works. The wonderful thing about a protein-centric approach is that the appetite tends to self-regulate once foods that unnaturally stimulate the appetite (such as processed sugar, grains and oils) are removed and the focus is on high-quality protein and other nutrients (mostly from animal sources). You can simply eat when you're hungry and stop when you're full the way we should!

DAY 4 CALORIE CONFUSION

We're all familiar with the concept of calories and the idea of "energy balance". While there is a "grain" of truth to this idea (no pun intended), it's overly simplistic and doesn't take into consideration that the macronutrient composition of the foods (along with other factors such as level of processing) determines their hormonal impact and what the body does with them.

When the energy balance hypothesis (calories in / calories out) was first proposed we had a very low level of understanding about obesity and most of the hormones that regulate appetite and energy expenditure hadn't even been discovered. Once we knew insulin, leptin, ghrelin and other hormones were affected differently by protein, fat and carbohydrates, meal-timing and other factors it was too late. The energy balance idea had already been entrenched in the public consciousness through repetition.

Yes, the amount of energy (calories) in foods is a major factor in achieving or maintaining a healthy weight and body composition but the TYPES of foods are way more important. Case in point, most ultra-processed foods are created to be overeaten and they have addictive properties by design.

On the other hand, it's virtually impossible to overeat a diet consisting mainly of lean protein and natural healthy sources of fat possibly along with some fiber. The bottom line is the level of processing affects the health impact of foods.

At each stage of human "progress" we've had to expend less and less energy in order to extract more from our food. At one point in human history, processing foods actually improved their nutrient-density. For example, cooking with fire enabled us to derive more nutrients. Fermentation extended the lifespan of food and increased beneficial bacteria it contained.

Eventually, we crossed a threshold, and now processing makes food more hyperpalatable while simultaneously increasing energy-density and reducing nutrient-density. Modern ultra-processed foods also have addictive properties that make it more difficult to control the amount we consume. This is all by design with maximum profit in mind.

Let's take a little journey through time and "follow in the footsteps of our ancestors" as we uncover the truth about how our primitive biology is reacting to our modern environment. Scientists tell us that Pre-Agricultural or "Paleolithic" cuisine was anything but lean and green, according to a 2021 study on the diets of our ancestors. For a good 2 million years, Homo sapiens and their ancestors dined heavily on meat, putting them at the top of the food chain. They consumed plants only sporadically when these foods were available in the wild.

A look through hundreds of previous studies on everything from modern human anatomy and physiology to measures of the isotopes inside ancient human bones and teeth suggests we were primarily apex predators until roughly 12,000 years ago. Would pre-agricultural era humans pass up some wild berries or other edible plants? No they wouldn't, and in my opinion, neither should you. Would they consume them year-round on a daily basis? No they wouldn't, and neither should you.

Remember there's no such thing as a "perfect" diet but following the cues from history will take us towards better health and a better understanding.

Note* some of the information in this chapter based on commentary from host of Peak Human Podcast and documentary film maker Brian Sanders. I've been a strong supporter of the Food Lies documentary (which is now near completion as a docuseries for Netflix) since Brian first came on my podcast to talk about it back in 2018. I'm looking forward to seeing him complete the project and blow the lid off the food industry practices and government policies that created the obesity epidemic. You can contact or support Brian at foodlies.org

DAY 5 BUILD AND BURN

Most "fitness influencers" have no idea what it's like to be overweight, tired and sluggish with no drive, existing day after day in a prison of a body you don't enjoy. They can't really advise you on what works because they've always been fit and healthy and don't know the realities of the lifestyle overhaul required to make these kinds of changes.

For them, anything will work. Even something as vague as " just eat less and move more" or "just track your calories". Mainstream advice never worked for me and a growing number of people are recognizing it doesn't work for them either but the good news is that it doesn't require iron will or discipline. You don't have to repeat the mantra "no pain no gain" and sweat it out in the gym ad nauseum.

If you've read my first book Live Like an Athlete, you already know that at my heaviest I weighed 254 lbs. At the time I was about 33% bodyfat (clinically obese) and beginning to suffer health problems as a result of my lifestyle. My doctor recommended that I might consider losing some weight as an alternative to medication but wasn't able to provide a plan for me to do so.

That's when I broke away from the pack. I did what few people would do if they found themselves in this situation. I took charge of my own health and began seriously researching and applying everything I could learn about how the body works, especially anything concerning diet and exercise. What I learned along the way to permanently losing over 75 pounds of unhealthy bodyfat and reversing the metabolic damage I had accumulated until that point is that it's easier than most people think. It's mostly environmental (not genetic as some medical professionals are now suggesting). It begins with the right mindset, then extends to making a few simple changes in your daily habits that add up over time.

When I show my weight loss before and after photos everyone asks "How long did it take?" The honest answer is that it has taken every day of my life since I made the decision to live a different way. At 254 lbs I was a metabolic disaster and a ticking time bomb. I had high blood pressure and was at risk for every lifestyle induced "disease" known to man. Ithasn't always been easy. I put in the time and effort at the gym every day using a combination of strength training and cardiovascular exercise but I don't have to suffer through it and neither do you.

The habits have become so automatic at this point I don't even think about it amymore, but at one time I was literally ADDICTED to processed food. The major change I made was prioritizing animal- sourced protein and being more conscious of reducing carbohydrate +fat (energy) especially from sugar, grains and "vegetable" oils.

With exercise and nutrition it's always "quality over quantity". When I was obese, I enjoyed working out and even hit the gym a few days a week but I didn't have a goal or result in mind (or a real deadline) and those key distinctions make all the difference.

Remember "Consistency always beats intensity". It may seem like you're getting nowhere at times but keep showing up and giving it your best effort and over time you'll look back and see how far you've come. Just understand that there is no finish line. Whatever changes you make have to be sustainable, otherwise what's the point?

If you have specific questions about how to get started or keep going, please reach out to me by direct message through the contact information I provide in this book. If you're already one of my clients and you're getting results from these methods, I recommend writing a review on my Amazon Author page or on any of my social media or content channels to inspire others. Together we can change the face of health in America and in the world!

DAY 6 THE PLANT PARADOX

One of my main criticisms of a vegan approach (beyond it not being adequate nutritionally or sustainable for humans) is that it's easily abused by the food manufacturing and marketing industry.

 For example, at first glance, someone might think a "vegan" cookie is a healthier option but if you examine the nutrition panel, you'll see it's filled with the most problematic ingredients just like any other cookie. All they did was remove the (MOST EXPENSIVE) ingredients: milk and eggs, which were the only source of any actual nutrients this product might have contained and thus extended the shelf life and increased their profit margin. This is what the food manufacturers are trying to do to our entire food supply!

Protein dilution is REAL and it has been on the rise since the inception of the original Dietary Guidelines for Americans. Plant-based ingredients like sugar, flour, grains and seed-oils, are substituted for real food (usually animal-based ingredients) which INCREASES the amount of a particular food needed to reach satiety as validated by the Protein Leverage Theory. Our need for protein is so strong that it exerts a tremendous amount of leverage over everything else we eat.

Humans will always overeat dietary fat and carbohydrates in an effort to obtain sufficient dietary protein when total protein in a particular food is low. When we focus on animal-sourced protein and strive to take in roughly 1g of protein per pound of bodyweight each day, we automatically eat less of everything else. This concept is the underlying scientific principle behind a concept known as Protein Leverage Theory.

This doesn't even take into account the inflammation, appetite dysregulation and other negative effects inherent in the aforementioned ingredients.

"Vegan" is a perfect example of what is known aa the "Halo Effect" in food labeling. The general public doesn't have time to evaluate everything they hear in the media regarding what's supposedly healthy, so most people just gravitate to what's popular or what they hear being promoted most often. Food manufacturers know this and often slap a trendy label on their packaging to entice buyers to temporarily override their innate discernment regarding processed foods by offering selections that are "Low Fat" or "Gluten Free" or other buzzwords.

The truth is that "plant-based" means nothing in terms of improving health. The most problematic ingredients sugar, flour and seed-oils are all plant-based! By vilifying animal-based ingredients, the food manufacturers simply create a demand for their supposedly healthier alternatives.

"Plant-based" is just the newest iteration of the low-fat idea that hurled the country headfirst into an epidemic of obesity and metabolic disorders. I'm not here to suggest we should just eat meat only and nothing else but the Carnivore Diet serves as evidence that it's possible to do this without suffering any negative health consequences.

The bottom line is there's no justification for reducing animal-based foods to improve health. Animal-based foods are high in nutrients and increasing their consumption usually improves overall health. Most of the negative health effects they supposedly have promoted by the popular media are based on epidemiological studies that involve dietary recall questionnaires and merely show correlation not causation. Every single published double-blind, randomized controlled trial shows higher protein and nutrients from animal sources has a positive impact on health outcomes. Even without scientific data, which is sometimes difficult to obtain because of bias on the part of researchers and difficulty obtaining funds for such research at the university level, there are thousands on anecdotal reports of people like me who have drastically improved our health and fitness by increasing not reducing their consumption of animal foods.

DAY 7 YOU ARE WHAT YOU EAT

In nature, a carnivore is defined as "an organism that eats meat or exclusively meat". Just as there are different types of carnivores there are different types of Carnivore diets. Let's take a quick look at the more popular ones.

The Lion Diet: This is the most restrictive version and includes only meat and organs of ruminant animals. Dr Shawn Baker and Mikhaila Peterson are notable advocates of this version of the diet.

Hypercarnivore: 70% or more of the foods consumed are animal sources. May also include fish, fowl, eggs and possibly some dairy.

Keto/Carnivore or Ketovore: Eliminates virtually all carbohydrate sources including those found in some starchy tubers and fruit. The emphasis on animal protein is the main difference between this and a clinical ketogenic diet. The emphasis is still on maintaining a state of ketosis. (Note* excess protein will get converted to glucose through a process known as gluconeogenesis. However, this will not kick you out of ketosis as many people believe because the process is demand-driven not supply-driven.)

Animal-Based: Mostly strict carnivore but includes plant sources of carbohydrates from honey and fruit. Dr Paul Saladino is the main promoter of this way of eating. This is touted as a more performance-based version of carnivore and is better suited to those not primarily seeking fat loss.

In all of its various forms, the carnivore diet is essentially an "elimination diet" so it's more about what you're avoiding than what you're eating. The main idea is once you reduce or eliminate low-nutrient, high calorie processed food-like products you're only left with a relatively small list of natural edible foods namely meat, fish, fowl, eggs, fruit, vegetables, fungi, nuts and seeds. Of those, the animal sources are higher in protein and other vital nutrients.

Humans are technically classified as omnivores because we eat from both the plant and animal kingdoms. I think the case could be made that we're "obligate carnivores" because we rely on the animal kingdom exclusively for at least some essential nutrients such as vitamin B-12.
On the other hand, there are no essential nutrients derived exclusively from plants. In fact, there isn't a single plant nutrient that isn't available from animal sources in a higher quality and more absorbable form.

I've personally witnessed several instances of people developing nutrient-deficiencies when attempting to eliminate all animal products from their diet (namely anemia or iron deficiency, protein deficiency leading to muscle wasting, low bone density and hair loss as well as B-12 deficiency.) This is not the case with reducing or eliminating most plants from the diet.

As a species, we have adapted to eating both plants and animals. Consumption of plants as a food source increased in the Agricultural Age when our health began to decline and further escalated in the Industrial Age when we developed full-blown epidemic of obesity and metabolic disorders. For most of human history animals were the primary food sources with only a small number of edible non-poisonous plants available and even that was highly seasonal. Plants have historically been "survival foods" to prevent starvation in the absence of animal-based nutrition if, for example, the herds of grazing ruminants had moved on or the hunting, fishing or trapping was unsuccessful that day.

As Apex predators, we are at the top of the food chain and have the ability to not only eat plants but also to eat other animals who can eat the plants for us, bioaccumulating and biomagnifying the nutrients in those plants into the most bioavalable forms!

One of my criticisms of the carnivore diet is the "all or nothing" mentality associated with it. You might think, as I did, that you can't just be a "little bit carnivore". You either eat nothing but meat or you don't. However, this is not true. Any increases in red meat and eggs or limiting of carbohydrates specifically from sugar and flour or processed grains is a step in the right direction in my opinion. If you just want to "ease into it" you can start by employing a "more of this, less of that" kind of thinking and see how you feel. If the result is positive, just continue heading in that direction. Who knows how far you could go?

DAY 8 CHEAT MEALS VS REFEEDS

To cheat or not to cheat? That is the question. While there is no structured "cheat day" on the 14 Day Carnivore Challenge I have always been a fan of it. I'd like to encourage you to stick around after this two week jump-start as we transition into a more sustainable lifetime program that allows for structured refeeds on the weekends.

When it comes to long-term adherence to nutritional and exercise principles, I use the 80/20 rule. This rule states that 80% of your results come from 20% of your efforts and vice versa. The other 80% of your activities only account for 20% of your results.

What are the "critical few" that you must do every single day to succeed in improving your health? Here's what I've learned along the way to losing 75 pounds and maintaining a new healthy weight for several years.

1) Exercise every day for 30-60 minutes minimum. Ideally this should be strength training followed by some cardiovascular activity. If you want to break them up into separate sessions, perform cardio in the morning on an empty stomach to prioritize fat-burning while in a semi-fasted state. Do your strength training later in the day after you have eaten something.

2) Drink at least 1/2 oz of water per lb of body weight daily.

3) Aim for 1-1.5 g of protein per lb of body weight day. Make it the focus of every meal and every snack.

4) Set goals. Write them down and track them relentlessly.

5) Take a day off or at least have one rest day or "cheat meal" every week. This is what will keep you in the game for the long run.

I know going back to your problem foods is the last thing you want to do right now but eventually you will learn how to fit them in without causing any damage. In fact, in the right context, a higher calorie or "junk food" meal is actually beneficial because it helps you psychologically stay in control of when and where it happens. You didn't "fail" if you indulged because it's part of the program! The all-or-nothing mindset is a recipe for disaster because no one can eat "perfectly" all the time forever so accept that when you do diverge it's not a reason to give up. Just start over again for another week.

The body adapts very quickly to a lower daily average amount of energy (calorie) intake and occasionally ramping up that amount helps keep the body in fat-burning, muscle building or muscle preservation mode. A carb-refeed is a nutritional strategy that allows you to eat more carbohydrates without storing them as fat! In fact, if you time it properly, they can actually improve metabolism, allowing you to build more muscle and burn bodyfat. This works best on a Keto/Carnivore or Ketovore Diet. (See Day 7 for details.)

Basically, you limit your carb intake during the week and only consume a significant amount of carbohydrates on the weekends (ideally in the evening and/or after a training session). At this time, you will have depleted muscle glycogen stores through your training efforts and improved your insulin sensitivity significantly. This causes incoming carbohydrates to be stored in the muscle tissue as glycogen rather than being stored as fat.

If you're skeptical about this method try it for yourself! Start each day with mainly animal-source protein along with some fat and very little carbohydrates, like eggs or whey protein or a little cream in your coffee for example. This will keep insulin low and allow you to burn bodyfat as energy more readily. Continue this pattern for five days until the end of the week when you'll have a "clean" portion of carbohydrate such as potatoes or rice. If you can time this to immediately follow a workout that's even better but it also works if you train in the morning.

As you progress, you can increase the amount and types of carbohydrates without experiencing any negative effects. The key is keeping your carbohydrate intake very low at all other times.

I've used this method to break a weight loss "plateau" and take my body to a new level of leanness. The effectiveness of this method is mainly due to the fact that increasing carbohydrates strategically improves leptin levels which prompts the body to release fat stores. Indulging in a higher calorie meal also gives you a break from the routine and allows you to indulge in some of your favorite foods which may not fit the animal-based, low-carb or ancestrally-appropriate template without causing any harm.

It's not realistic or sustainable long-term to think you will never diverge from your way of eating. Having an opportunity to take a break without losing ground makes the method I'm suggesting more of a lifestyle and less of a "diet". I want to help people like you learn to follow a way of eating and exercising that you can continue for five, ten even twenty years or more from now. In contrast most people think of a diet as a temporary restriction they only have to do for a brief time until they reach their goal. This is not practical for most. My hope is that you learn new habits you can maintain for a lifetime!

DAY 9 GET IN THE ZONE

It's the start of another week and today is a rest day but beginning tomorrow many of us will be hitting the gym over the next few days in hopes of undoing our dietary indiscretions over the weekend. Every major holiday is followed by droves of gymgoers attempting to outrun their environment (and genetics) by hitting everyone's favorite torture device, the treadmill!

If you subscribe to the energy-balance or "calories-in / calories-out" theory of weight loss it makes perfect sense to exercise at a higher intensity level and therefore "burn more calories" which will increase a calorie deficit and result in burning more bodyfat. However, this is not an accurate model of human metabolism and many well-intentioned people have been severely disappointed with their results despite an honest effort while attempting to employ this method.

In nature, humans are classified as "persistence hunters" and our ability to outlast (not outrun) every other species on the planet is what ensured our survival for thousands of years. The old saying "slow and steady wins the race" is also true when it comes to the greatest modern threats to human existence; metabolic syndrome and obesity.

Understanding how "low and slow cardio" is more effective at burning stored bodyfat than high-intensity effort requires a little basic understanding of human physiology. There are various "pathways" the body utilizes to produce energy and they vary based on the demand. The first few seconds of high intensity activity are fueled by the phosphagen system which is depleted rapidly, within about 15 seconds. This is the energy system used for lifting weights or strength training activities and is only available briefly before taking a rest period to regenerate ATP.

Cardiovascular activity can be either aerobic or anaerobic in nature. That means it relies on oxygen or it doesn't. At more moderate intensity levels we remain in the aerobic zone producing most of the energy required primarily from stored bodyfat.

When the intensity exceeds a certain level and the body can no longer break down fat fast enough to keep up with the energy demand, we switch over to the glycolytic pathway which requires the breakdown of glucose for energy. Glucose a.k.a "sugar" is stored in the muscles as glycogen so some of the glucose required for brief sprints or muscle-building activity taking longer than 15 seconds can be derived from this source and replaced at the next meal and it's no big deal.

Remember, even if you don't eat carbohydrates frequently your body can break down protein through the process of gluconeogenesis to refill these stores.

Beyond the first few seconds of high intensity activity, we switch over from lipolysis (fat-burning) to glycolysis (sugar-burning) and if you're eating low carb and performing strength training on an almost daily basis the way I recommend, your stores of glycogen won't be topped off and your body will actually begin catabolizing or breaking down muscle and turning it into glucose. This is not an ideal scenario. We always want to preserve or add muscle to keep metabolic function high.

Furthermore, the body sees all of this energy-demanding muscle as a liability if you're running for your life all the time, especially if it perceives a shortage of dietary energy in the environment because you're eating less carbs and fat, eating smaller portions or eating less frequently. To ensure survival, and improve your ability to train at a high-intensity level without burning tons of energy that aren't being replenished often enough, your body will dump some of that muscle which will cause you to lose weight but will also make you weaker, less healthy and less resilient throughout life.

To stay in the fat burning "zone" aim for a target heart rate of 180 minus your age. That's the B.P.M. (beats per minute) where you can still derive most of the energy needed from fat. Most cardiovascular exercise equipment has some type of built in heart rate sensor. If you're training outdoors or on a machine that isn't equipped with this feature, you can measure your pulse rate and estimate your BPM on that. You can also train at a level of intensity that makes it slightly difficult to breathe but not impossible to carry on a conversation. This is where you want to be to derive most of the energy required to support the activity from your fat stores not your hard-earned and metabolically invaluable muscle.

Further perpetuating the problem, high intensity activity makes you hungry (for glucose) and consequently may cause you to overeat after a workout. I see this pattern all the time. People eat sugar, burn sugar, then eat more sugar. They never get around to burning fat as they intended because they have plenty of glucose in the bloodstream or stored in the body.

Carbohydrate basically "gets in the way" of fat-burning and the solution is to reduce your overall carbohydrate intake in total amount, frequency or both. That gives the body a chance to tap into stored energy, which is the reason we have stored bodyfat in the first place! Give this technique a try. You just may be amazed at how easy it is to get results by not filling your body with glucose that you have to burn so you don't store it as fat in the first place. The additional benefit of utilizing a less physically-demanding form of training may also cause you to breathe a sigh of relief. Your body will thank you!

DAY 10 THE SCIENCE OF ANCESTRAL DIETS

Diet trends come and go, but the one that has stood the test of time in some form or another is the Low Carbohydrate Diet. The Low Carbohydrate (or low carb) way of eating has actually been around for thousands of years! What other diet can make that claim?

Scientists believe our ancestors ate a diet that consisted primarily of meat, fish, eggs, fowl and some nuts and seeds. Fruit and tubers were hard to come by (except seasonally) and most modern vegetables didn't even exist for the majority of human history. Our troubles really began when we learned how to domesticate animals and started cultivating plants for food. This crisis further escalated in modern times thanks to industrialization and later with mass processing and distribution of high carb, low nutrient foods. Low-carb diets have been gaining popularity recently due to the simple fact that they work! The reasons for this are fairly simple.

For starters, most of the foods people tend to overeat often contain large amounts of carbohydrates, (mainly from highly refined ingredients such as sugar and flour). Due to their sheer volume in the food supply, these are the most likely sources of calories to be eaten in excess and therefore stored as bodyfat.

Secondly, carbohydrates suppress the burning of fat (our body's natural fuel source) because excess glucose is toxic to humans it must be burned first when it is present in the bloodstream. Only when glucose has been used as energy or stored for later can the body return to its default fat-burning state.

The body maintains a very small and very tightly controlled amount of glucose at all times and anything over about a teaspoon has to be burned immediately or shuttled into storage before it starts causing damage. In order to dispose of the extra glucose (or blood sugar) insulin is dispatched.

When insulin is elevated, fat burning screeches to a halt. In short bursts insulin is not problematic. In fact, we would die without it. It's only when insulin levels are chronically elevated that it becomes a problem. In fact, chronically elevated insulin (hyperinsulinemia as the condition is known) is the root cause of metabolic disorders we're experiencing as a society. The solution is replacing the majority of empty calories we consume from carbohydrates with quality sources of nutrients like protein and essential fats. The bottom line is EAT REAL FOOD.

The so-called "carnivore" diet originally began as an attempt by biohackers and others interested in optimizing their health to emulate a "zero carb" way of eating that was also higher in dietary protein compared to a clinical ketogenic diet. (The original clinical keto diet was designed to mimic the effects of fasting to prevent seizures in epileptic children.) Once it was discovered to have weight-loss benefits as well, news spread about this exciting "new" way of eating. Again, it was only a new concept to the general public although the bodybuilding community had been utilizing this approach for decades.

As early as the 1950's Bodybuilding pioneer Vince Gironda devised a style of eating known as the "steak and eggs diet". This was essentially an animal-based, low-carb/ketogenic diet with carb refeeds or cheat meals on the weekends.

In the 1980's another contribution was made by Dr. Mauro DiPasquale who called his plan "The Anabolic Diet". Dr. DiPasquale was a bodybuilder and strength athlete who also coached others in the sport. He popularized the term "cyclical ketogenic diet" to describe his nutritional protocol which is very similar to the "steak and eggs" method. With its high reliance on animal protein and general avoidance of carbohydrates five days a week, and a high-carbohydrate phase on the weekends his Anabolic Diet soon became popular with a new generation of fitness enthusiasts. He went on to publish his results in the pages of various powerlifting and musclebuilding magazines, newsletters and books.

Out of necessity, the "in-the-trenches" implementation of this lifestyle led bodybuilders and other fitness enthusiasts to recognize the need for higher dietary protein intake to build and-or maintain muscle. As a historical reference, adherents cite entire populations such as the Inuit who regularly went extended periods of time with zero dietary carbohydrate and still enjoyed wonderful health.

In summary, while this approach may sound radical and extreme it has a rich history of being used safely and effectively.

DAY 11 FAT FOR FUEL

Do you want to know a secret? Burning fat is our default state! Our bodies are designed to use stored fat as energy when there is no food available. That's why we don't die from starvation while we sleep each night. We only interrupt this process by consuming a competing form of energy produced mainly from carbohydrates called glucose or blood sugar.

You can think of your body as a "hybrid engine" that can also use glucose as fuel when present or in times of increased demand. If we're trying to "run for our lives' as in an all-out sprint or similar endeavor, that activity is 100% fueled by sugar (glucose). Because we always need some glycogen (stored glucose) on hand "just in case" we can even convert protein into glycogen to refill our tank for emergency use.

Metabolic Flexibility (the ability to shift back and forth and combust various forms of fuel to meet our energy demands) is something many of us have lost, thanks to a constant barrage of carbohydrates, eaten very frequently, over a long period of time. If continued, this pattern eventually leads to insulin resistance and if left unchecked, Type 2 or "adult onset" diabetes. I'll go over this in more detail in the final chapter of this book.

One of the major keys to improving insulin sensitivity and restoring your innate ability to run on fat is to reduce carbohydrate intake either in amount, frequency, or both. This method, when combines with strength training and cardiovascular Activity produces unparalleled results.

How did we get the idea that carbohydrates are so great in the first place? Much of this has to do with the massive disinformation campaign we've all been subjected to for years. In layman's terms it's "marketing". There is big money tied up in high glucose-producing grains and refined sweeteners. Far from the "preferred fuel" that it's purported to be, glucose is actually toxic in high amounts in the bloodstream. Therefore, it must be cleared before we can resume our default fat-burning state.

In our "hybrid engine" analogy you can think of glucose as gasoline and fat as battery power. We only switch over to burning fat when the gas tank gets low. In an all-out sprint, we rely almost exclusively on glucose to fuel the activity. Most of us in the modern world never do anything remotely resembling an all-out sprint. We're also constantly topping off the fuel tank even when it's already full. The result is the unused energy is simply converted to bodyfat and stored in the adipose tissue for later use.

In order to clear glucose, insulin is dispatched to drive it either into the muscle cells to fuel activity or be stored as glycogen for future use or else into fat cells for the same purpose. When we constantly overwhelm our body, the cells become insulin resistant. Eventually, rising glucose levels get high enough to be classified as Type 2 (aka adult onset) Diabetes. Sadly, this condition is now becoming more common among children.

The late great Dr. Robert C Atkins, a true pioneer in low-carb nutrition, said it best "If you want to burn fat, remove the fuel that burns before fat." He was referring, of course, to carbohydrates. I don't want to give the impression that I believe any and all carbohydrate sources are to be avoided at all times. Our hunter-gatherer ancestors would have occasionally stumbled across some ripe fruit in season, a hive containing honey or the occasional tuber like a potato, for example, and taken advantage of this opportunity. I believe we should enjoy these types of foods as well, just less frequently and in smaller amounts. This is why I'm known for saying "we can eat *whatever* we want, just not *whenever* we want. Nutrient timing is also a critical factor that rarely gets discussed by the mostly sedentary population. To an athlete or fitness enthusiast, nutrition is critical and the cycle of "prepare and repair" is a twenty-four hour daily reality.

DAY 12 HOW DOES A CARNIVORE DIET WORK?

For decades the so-called "experts" have been telling us to avoid the healthiest foods on the planet (primarly, meat, eggs and other animal-based goodies) and instead to eat cheap, processed garbage (mainly sugar, processed grains and industrial seed oils). Why?

Could it be the policy-makers and their corporate cronies want to maximize their profits and allow us to be weak, sick and basically dependant on pharmaceutical drugs so they can control us more easily?
It's time to wake up and take back control of your own health!

It theory any style of eating that causes you to consume less dietary energy than you expend will result in weight loss. However, "weight loss" and body composition are two entirely different things. The target of this program (and any program aimed at improving metabolic health) should be to reduce excess bodyfat while maintaining or adding muscle. The bottom line is the more muscle and less fat you have, the better you will look, feel and perform in everything you do.

The underlying factors that cause a carnivore diet to be effective at accomplishing this are the following:
1) It is adequate in complete protein which contains all the necessary raw materials that our muscles (as well as hair, skin, nails, joints bones and organs) are made of in the most bioavailable form.

2) It supplies all of the necessary essential fats, especially Omega 3 fatty acids that promote heart and brain health while lowering systemic inflammation.

3) It is inherently low in carbohydrates since they aren't abundant in animal foods and therefore it doesn't contain "empty calories" from a source that wreaks havoc on appetite, sabotages our energy and overrides our best intentions at self-control, especially when consumed in higher amounts.

While you may achieve the coveted state of a "calorie deficit" by reducing calories from fat or carbohydrates, in my experience, a low-carb diet is easier to adhere to than a low-fat diet because it reduces hunger by blunting insulin and allows the body to access fat as fuel more easily. This also explains why The Standard American Diet based on the Dietary Guidelines for Americans has been an unmitigated failure.

I feel that prioritizing protein is really the key to sustainable success on a Carnivore diet (or any diet for that matter). This is true because of these facts about protein:

1) Protein has the highest thermic effect of any micronutrient, meaning it takes more energy to process, store and assimilate than any other macronutrient.

2) Protein provides the highest level of satiety which curbs cravings. Satiety is just a fancy word for the satisfaction you get from a filling meal. This is important for long-term adherence. In theory you can lose weight by simply reducing "calories" across the board but how likely would you be to stick to a low-satiety way of eating long term?

3) Protein helps build or maintain lean mass which is the ultimate driver of metabolic rate. The more muscle you have, the more energy your body requires around the clock.

Don't let anyone fool you into thinking that a low-carb, animal-based way of eating doesn't taste good or it's "boring". Plant-,based ingredients like wheat and other grains are about the most bland thing I could imagine eating! On the other hand, meat and other animal foods are delicious when prepared properly and can be used in a variety of dishes to suit a variety of tastes.

If I had to summarize my advice into a simple slogan that would be easy to remember and to put into action, it would be "Eat Meat Not Wheat". Our health crisis escalated because we were deceived into thinking we should avoid meat (and other animal-based foods) and instead we should eat wheat (and other grains like corn, oats and rice). The solution is to do the exact opposite of what the authorities recommend!

DAY 13 SLOW POISON

Processed foods (mostly containing some combination of sugar, flour and industrial seed oils aka "vegetable" oils) are at the heart of the obesity problem and metabolic syndrome. They ruin our health, then pharmaceutical drugs are offered as a remedy for the ill effects. The root problem is never addressed by most doctors and the cycle continues. This, by the way, is why it's called the Food AND Drug Administration. One corrupt government entity oversees the whole mess, and we "pay the price" often at the expense of our own health.

The idea that we can simply eat smaller amounts of the offending ingredients (known as the calorie-centric approach) is doomed to fail because these foods are designed to be addictive and provide almost pure energy from carbs and fat with no actual nutrients. These are the things to reduce or eliminate from the diet as much as possible.

It is now well-known that the multibillion-dollar food manufacturing companies employ scientists to run test groups to determine the exact amount of an ingredient (like sugar for example) needed to reach what is known as the "bliss point" and elicit an addictive response that causes people to eat uncontrollably.

How can we identify the problem foods? Here's a hint: If it couldn't even exist without the use of industrial machinery, it's a processed food. It's not necessary to go all the way back to the Stone Age to see where it all went wrong. People were generally healthy, and obesity was virtually non-existent just 50-100 years ago, before the advancements in food processing and other technology made the mass-production, marketing and distribution of junk food possible.

If there is a "ground zero" for the obesity epidemic, it would be the implementation of the original Dietary Guidelines for Americans that told the population to ditch foods high in saturated fat like meat and eggs and instead to eat grains and industrial seed oils.

This turned out to be a major mistake and to this day by the admission of the USDA themselves "The Dietary Guidelines have never been specifically tested for health benefits!" It was all promoted for financial reasons and nothing more since day one.

Now that we have identified the problem as foods high in energy and low in nutrients, the solution is clear. Concentrate instead on nutrients like protein, fiber and EFA's found in real food. The list of those is pretty concise: Meat, Fish, Eggs, Vegetables, Nuts, Seeds and Fruit. If you have problems metabolizing even natural sugar, stay with low-sugar fruit like olives or avocado and eliminate starchy tubers and root vegetables as well.

If you want to hit the "bullseye" of human nutrition, limit your foods to the most nutrient-dense choices such as red meat and eggs, then limit all plant foods including even vegetables. I don't think vegetables are harmful to our health but their nutrient value has been vastly overstated and in order to make them appealing most people cover them in unhealthy oils from commercial salad dressings or add high calorie-density ingredients.

Remember, quality beats quantity every single time. This is the philosophy behind Ancestral Health Principles and specifically dietary strategies like Paleo, Keto and Carnivore. When the quality of food is high the quantity tends to take care of itself. It's usually only necessary to meticulously track every gram that goes into our mouth when we're trying to fit in too many ultra processed foods. I'll explain the "bullseye" concept along with a diagnostic tool I created called the Carb Sensitivity Spectrum in more detail over the next two days as we wrap up the challenge.

DAY 14 THE REAL HUMAN DIET

We made it! Now that the 14 Day Carnivore Challenge is over it's time to think about where to go next from here. As I stated earlier in this book, the Carnivore Diet is essentially an "elimination diet". That means it's aimed at improving your way of eating by eliminating certain foods or categories of foods that may be problematic for you. In the case of the Carnivore Diet that would be plant material.

Our society thrives on the extreme approach and a true Carnivore Diet consisting of nothing more than meat, salt and water would definitely fit that bill! I don't personally follow a strict carnivore approach, nor do I recommend it to anyone. I wrote this book as a reference for those who are curious about this method and simply to have a reason to research it more thoroughly.

That being said, my personal experience of losing 75 pounds of bodyfat that I have maintained for several years, combined with the successes of others that I've helped to create through my coaching programs, have led me to believe there is merit in reducing at least some plant material from the diet, beginning with the worst examples of "technology gone wild"; sugar, flour/processed grains and industrial seed oils aka "vegetable" oil.

Being of plant origin is not what makes these ingredients harmful. It's the fact that they represent sources of pure refined dietary energy with little or no nutritional value. In other words, they are "empty calories". Additionally, these ingredients promote inflammation, appetite-dysregulation and other negative effects that will prevent you from reaching your optimal state of health and fitness or at least make it more difficult to achieve.

Another valuable principle of a carnivore diet is that it focuses on real food, especially the (arguably most nutrient-dense ones that are all of animal origin). Real food doesn't have labels. PRODUCTS have labels. The one thing the adherents to the various Ancestral Health diets like Paleo, Keto and Carnivore agree on is that processed "food" is the heart of the problem. Even a strict Vegan wouldn't argue with that.

Everyone is unique in their preferences but don't be fooled by slick marketing. About 80% of what is sold in stores is not real food. You've heard to "shop the perimeter" of the grocery store right? Think about what is out there. Meat, seafood, eggs, dairy and produce. What's in the center aisles? Mostly grains, sugar, flour, Industrial seed oils, corn syrup and other processed food products.

I have developed a Carb-Sensitivity-Spectrum Questionairre that I can't print in its entirety at this time, but briefly ask yourself what effect does consuming a high carbohydrate meal or snack have on the following:

1 Energy (Is it sluggish or do you feel "ready to go"?)
2 Appetite (Especially three or four hours later. This is a sure sign of the energy roller-coaster due to insulin spikes and crashes that many people experience as a daily reality)
3 Mood (Do you get "hangry" if you miss a meal? Do you get shaky or feel weak without frequently consuming carbohydrates? These are keys to revealing your level of glucose-dependency.) Not being able to last more

than a few hours without a snack is a very vulnerable and weak metabolic state to be in.

4 Fasted Glucose, A1C (or other blood markers)

Depending on your score you might chose the real food route that allows you to have a Significant Carbohydrate Load *SCL on the following scale:

Every 4-6 hours (Paleo / Carb-Backloading)

Every 4-6 days (Carb Cycling or Cyclical Ketogenic Diet)

Every 4-6 weeks (Zero Carb Carnivore or Ketovore Diet

The major concept I want readers to take away from this book is the understanding that a lifestyle including weight training, some regular cardiovascular activity and a high-protein, low-carb way of eating creates more storage space in the muscle and liver to buffer incoming glucose and also increases insulin sensitivity in the muscle tissue.

After a week of this protocol the muscles are hungry for carbohydrates. Stick around for my next book that continues to explore resistance exercise low-carb/ ketogenic diets and Intermittent fasting through an ancestral lens. Subscribe by email or follow my social media and other content at linktr.ee/truetransformation.coach As always, I welcome your comments below and until next time stay strong and enjoy the journey! – Jason .

ABOUT THE AUTHOR

Jason Atkinson is a certified health coach and personal trainer who lost 75 pounds of bodyfat and reversed his symptoms of metabolic syndrome using an Ancestral approach that he is passionate about communicating. For more content or to become a client visit linktr.ee/truetransformation.coach.

Made in the USA
Columbia, SC
04 September 2023

22468970R00038